AF646174

Cumulative Student Activity Record of Clinical Experience
for
Post Basic BSc Nursing Program
(Log Book)

Prepared as per Syllabus of INC New Delhi and BFUHS Faridkot (Punjab)

Cumulative Student Activity Record of Clinical Experience for Post Basic Bsc Nursing Program (Log Book)

HC Rawat
Vice-Principal
University College of Nursing
Baba Farid University of Health Sciences
Faridkot, Punjab, India

Navdeep Kaur Brar
Senior Demonstrator
University College of Nursing
Baba Farid University of Health Sciences
Faridkot, Punjab, India

Foreword
SS Gill

University College of Nursing
Baba Farid University of Health Sciences
Faridkot – 151203 Punjab, India

JAYPEE BROTHERS MEDICAL PUBLISHERS (P) LTD

New Delhi • Panama City • London • Dhaka • Kathmandu

Jaypee Brothers Medical Publishers (P) Ltd

Headquarters

Jaypee Brothers Medical Publishers (P) Ltd
4838/24, Ansari Road, Daryaganj
New Delhi 110 002, India
Phone: +91-11-43574357
Fax: +91-11-43574314
Email: jaypee@jaypeebrothers.com

Overseas Offices

J.P. Medical Ltd
83, Victoria Street, London
SW1H 0HW (UK)
Phone: +44-2031708910
Fax: +02-03-0086180
Email: info@jpmedpub.com

Jaypee-Highlights Medical Publishers Inc.
City of Knowledge, Bld. 237, Clayton
Panama City, Panama
Phone: +507-301-0496
Fax: +507-301-0499
Email: cservice@jphmedical.com

Jaypee Brothers Medical Publishers (P) Ltd
17/1-B Babar Road, Block-B, Shaymali
Mohammadpur, Dhaka-1207
Bangladesh
Mobile: +08801912003485
Email: jaypeedhaka@gmail.com

Jaypee Brothers Medical Publishers (P) Ltd
Shorakhute, Kathmandu
Nepal
Phone: +00977-9841528578
Email: jaypee.nepal@gmail.com

Website: www.jaypeebrothers.com
Website: www.jaypeedigital.com

Inquiries for bulk sales may be solicited at: jaypee@jaypeebrothers.com

Cumulative Student Activity Record of Clinical Experience for Post Basic BSc Nursing Program

First Edition: **2013,** Reprint: 2026

ISBN: 978-93-5090-405-3

Typeset at: JPBMP typesetting unit

Printed in India

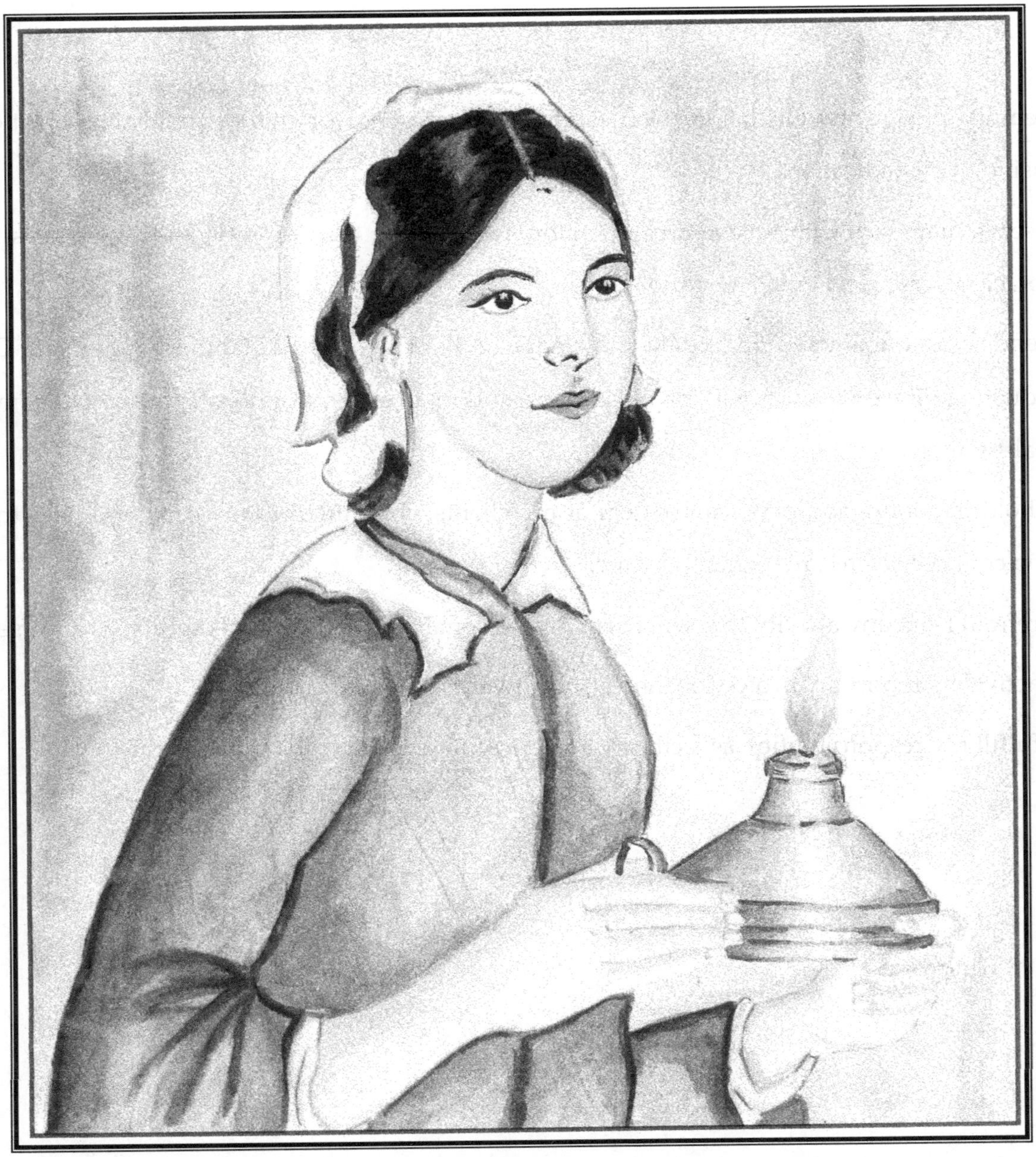

Miss Florence Nightingale

"A Lady with the Lamp"

Born on: May 12th, 1820

Died on : August 13th, 1910

Nurse's Pledge

"I solemnly pledge myself, before God, and in the presence of this assembly, to practice my profession, with dedication.

I will serve mankind, with love and compassion, recognizing their dignity, and rights irrespective of color, caste, creed, religion and nationality.

I will endeavor to maintain, up-to-date knowledge and skill to uphold standard of Nursing Care to individual, family and community, in all settings, and in all aspects of holistic care, as a member of the health care team.

I will hold in confidence, personal matters of my clients, committed to my care, and help them to develop confidence, in care rendered by me.

I will refrain from any activity that will harm my personal and professional dignity, as a nurse.

I will actively support my profession, and strive towards its advancement.

I will fulfill my responsibilities, as a citizen, and encourage change, to optimum care."

Preface

Nursing is a profession demanding nurses to have proper acquisition of three domains of education i.e. cognitive, psychomotor, communicative skills. Psychomotor domain is the skill to practice various nursing procedures. It is a vital components in clinical practice which need adequate knowledge and perfection in performing skills/procedures and repeated practices. Clinical activities mentioned in this record book are minimum requirement to obtain Post Basic BSc Nursing degree.

The core activities of clinical experience is that a student will be able to understand, comprehend and correlate the theoretical knowledge with practice and develop various skills based on scientific principles in performing a number of clinical activities related to nursing.

The main purpose of this clinical activities record is to explore that the various nursing procedures/skills have been demonstrated/taught by nursing faculty and practiced by students with expected level of satisfaction to provide quality nursing care to the individual, community, etc. Independently in their future.

This record book will help students to appreciate the patients as a holistic individual and develop skill to function as a trained nurse. It will provide uniform learning opportunity regarding practices experienced by the student nurse under strict clinical supervision during the course.

This cumulative clinical activities record book is designed according to new syllabus approved by INC and Faculty of Nursing Sciences, Baba Farid University of Health Sciences, Faridkot, Punjab for Post Basic BSc Nursing Course.

HC Rawat

Foreword

The nursing colleges running under the state of Punjab were previously affiliated to different universities of Punjab. Since 1999, all the colleges clubbed together and know they are affiliated to Baba Farid University of Health Sciences, Faridkot, Punjab, in order to bring about uniformity in course contents, teaching methods and examination evaluation system which is based on INC, University curriculum and the recommendations of the nursing board of the study. The faculty members of the University College of Nursing (constituent college of Baba Farid University of Health Sciences, Faridkot) strongly felt need of developing an effective, comprehensive and cumulative clinical activity record to supplement revised curriculum to enhance clinical skills among nursing trainees. I am happy that this book for recording cumulative experiences, prepared by Prof HC Rawat and NK Brar, University College of Nursing with support of faculty members of University College of Nursing, as per the regulations of Indian Nursing Council and the revised curriculum of Baba Farid University of Health Sciences, Faridkot.

Every nursing college must recognize the importance of skillful clinical practical training and progress made by the student throughout the course. I think this record book will help in developing skills and build working confidence during performance of procedures in the clinical areas. This record book will provide useful information even for appointing examiners in the field of nursing. It helps in evaluation regarding the practical experience gained by the individual nurse trainee during the course. I am sure this record book which is comprehensive in its nature shall be well appreciated by the nursing students, demonstrators as well as faculty members of Baba Farid University of Health Sciences.

Prof (Dr) SS Gill
Vice Chancellor
BFUHS, Faridkot (Punjab)

Student's Identification Profile

Paste
Passport
Size Photograph

Name of the Student : ______________________

(In Capital Letters)

Father's Name : ______________________

Registration No : ______________________

Date of Birth : ______________________

Date of Joining the Course : ______________________

Date of Completion the Course: ______________________

Permanent Address : ______________________

____

____

____

Telephone Number : ______________ **E-mail:** ______________________

____

Signature of Student

Date

____

Signature of the Principal

Date

College Seal

General Objectives

During the clinical postings in the various areas of general specialities, nursing students will be able to understand, comprehend and develop skills in performing the various nursing procedures, strictly following the related scientific principles and rationales for every step adopted.

Contributory Objectives

During the clinical postings, the students will be able to:

1. Correlate theory with the clinical practice.
2. Acquire skills and the techniques of nursing procedures in clinical settings.
3. Correlate the knowledge from other disciplines while performing the steps of procedures.
4. Use systematic approach in performing the procedures.
5. Assemble and check the equipment required for the procedure.
6. Demonstrate the skills in performing the procedures accurately based on scientific principles.
7. Develop skills in assessing, planning, implementing and evaluating the nursing care in different set-ups, i.e. hospital and community.
8. Assess the learning needs of clients, plan and implement the health education.
9. Develop ability in documentation-reporting accurately and promptly.

Instructions for Proper use of Clinical Record Book

1. Make it sure that the student nurse has been instructed in the various types of nursing procedures and to record whether or not he/she has performed the procedure to the satisfaction of clinical instructor.
2. Entries should be made regularly and with care. The students record sheet should be marked every week after discussion with the students.
3. It is desirable that all procedures should be demonstrated in classroom before they are carried out in wards/clinical areas.
4. All procedures to be signed when the student has done it satisfactory in the classroom as well as in the ward, by the respective clinical instructors/demonstrators. In some cases where this is not possible, the procedure is signed after return-demonstration in the demonstration room only. In such cases the clinical instructors/demonstrators should indicate this by writing DR after her signature with a circle around the DR.
5. No student should be permitted to do any procedure independently unless he/she has obtained a signature for that procedure.
6. Procedures are to be signed after sufficient practice in the clinical areas.
7. The student is expected to take the responsibility for his/her learning by:
    a. Requesting the clinical instructor/demonstrator to supervise a procedure he/she is performing to have a signature.
    b. Volunteering for experience he/she needs.
    c. Taking the responsibility for obtaining a signature from clinical instructor/demonstrator who has supervised the procedure, immediately following the successful completion of the procedure.
8. Evaluation of student's performance should be carried out periodically.
9. A student must have all the procedures signed to be eligible for vivavoce and practical examination for each year and should present the same to the examiners.
10. Students must ensure that they get signatures from Internal and External examiners after completion of practical examination every year.

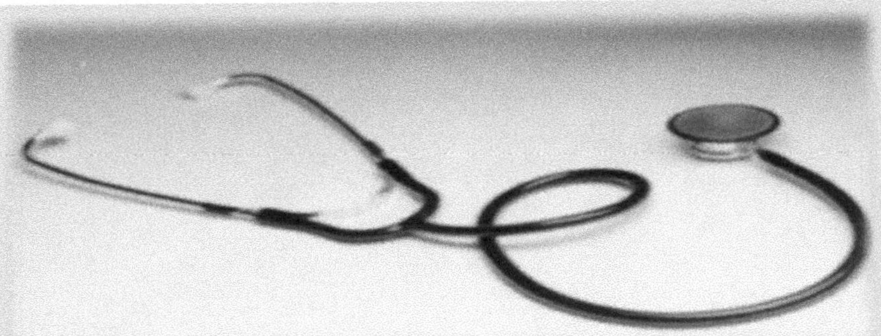

Ist Year Post Basic BSc (Nursing)

Hours of Instruction

Theory: Clinical Experience:

S No	Subjects	Theory (Hours)	Practical (Hours)
1	Nursing Foundation	45	–
2	Nutrition and Dietetics	30	15
3	Biochemistry and Biophysics	60	15
4	Psychology	60	–
5	Maternal Nursing	60	240
6	Child Health Nursing	60	240
7	Microbiology	60	30
8	Medical Surgical Nursing	60	270
9	English (Qualifying)	60	–
	Total Hours	**525**	**180**
	Total Hours	**705 hours**	

Subjects and Marks Distributions for Internal Assessment and University Examinations

S No	Subjects	Hours	Internal Assessment	University Exam	Total
1	Nursing Foundation	2	15	35	50
2	Nutrition and Dietetics	2	15	35	50
3	Biochemistry and Biophysics	3	25	75	100
4	Psychology	3	25	75	100
5	Microbiology	3	25	75	100
6	Maternal Nursing	3	25	75	100
7	Child Health Nursing	3	25	75	100
8	Medical Surgical Nursing	3	25	75	100
9	English	3	25	75	100
	Practical and Viva Voce				
	• Maternal Nursing		50	50	100
	• Child Health Nursing		50	50	100
	• Medical Surgical Nursing		50	50	100

Maternal Nursing

S No	Nursing Procedures	Lab Demonstration by Demonstrator		Clinical Demonstration by Student (Verified by Demonstrator)		Remarks
		Date	Signature	Date	Signature	
1	**Prenatal Care**					
	(a) Prenatal Assessment					
	(b) Prenatal Health Advice • Nutrition • Immunization • Exercise • Care of Breast					
	(c) Preparation for Non Stress Test and Ultrasound					
2	**Intranatal Care**					
	(a) Preparation for Delivery					
	(b) Setting up of Newborn Resuscitation Trolley					
	(c) Perineal Preparation for Labour					
	(d) Partogram					
	(e) PV Examination					
	(f) Normal Delivery					
	(g) Episiotomy and Suturing					
	(h) Apgar Scoring					
	(i) Newborn Assessment					

S No	Nursing Procedures	Lab Demonstration by Demonstrator		Clinical Demonstration by Student (Verified by Demonstrator)		Remarks
		Date	Signature	Date	Signature	
3	**Postnatal Care**					
	(a) Postnatal Care					
	(b) Postnatal Assessment					
	(c) Perineal Light					
	(d) Breast Care					
	(e) Assisting with Breastfeeding					
	(f) Postnatal Health Advice					
4	**Newborn Care**					
	(a) Assessment of Newborn					
	(b) Care of Normal Newborn					
	(c) Care of Baby in Ventilator					
	(d) Mummification					
	(e) Care of High-risk Newborn					
5	**Family Welfare**					
	(a) Motivation of Planned Parenthood					
	(b) Assist/Perform IUCD Insertion					

S No	Nursing Procedures	Lab Demonstration by Demonstrator		Clinical Demonstration by Student (Verified by Demonstrator)		Remarks
		Date	Signature	Date	Signature	
	(c) Assist/Observe Tubectomy					
	(d) Assist/Observe Vasectomy					
	Requirements					
	Antenatal Examinations- 20					
	Postnatal Examinations- 20					
	Per Vaginal Examinations- 20					
	Conducts Normal Delivery- 20					
	Motivation of Planned Parenthood-10					
	Stitching of Episiotomy- 20					
	Witness Caesarean Section- 10					

Practical File Work

1 Case Study	Date	Disease Condition	Signature
(a)			
(b)			
2 Nursing Care Plan			
(a)			
(b)			
(c)			
3 Health Talk			
(a)			
(b)			

Practical Examination

Signature of Internal Examiner

Date:

Signature of External Examiner

Date:

Signature of Internal Examiner

Date:

Signature of External Examiner

Date:

Child Health Nursing

S No	Nursing Procedures	Lab Demonstration by Demonstrator		Clinical Demonstration by Student (Verified by Demonstrator)		Remarks
		Date	Signature	Date	Signature	
1	Admission/Discharge of Children					
2	History Taking					
3	Physical Assessment • Newborn • Infant • Sick Child					
4	Calculation of Medicine Doses					
5	**Administration of Medication**					
	(a) Oral					
	(b) IM					
	(c) IV					
	(d) SC					
6	Preparation/Administration of ORS					
7	Calculation of IV Fluid Drop Rate/Dose					
8	Fluid Preparation (N/5, N/4, N/3, N/2) in 5% or 10% Dextrose					

S No	Nursing Procedures	Lab Demonstration by Demonstrator		Clinical Demonstration by Student (Verified by Demonstrator)		Remarks
		Date	Signature	Date	Signature	
9	**Collection of Specimen**					
	(a) Urine					
	(b) Blood					
	(c) Throat Swabs					
10	Methods of Oxygen Administration in Children					
11	**Nutritional Needs**					
	(a) Assist in Breastfeeding					
	(b) Paladie and Katori Feeding					
	(c) Nasogastric Feeding					
	(d) Gastrostomy Feeding					
	(e) Jejunostomy Feeding					
12	**Planning for Special Diet**					
	(a) PEM					
	(b) Nephrotic Syndrome					
	(c) Hepatic Encephalopathy					
	(d) Renal Failure					
13	**Care of Child In/On**					
	(a) Radiant Warmer					
	(b) Incubator					
	(c) Ventilator					

S No	Nursing Procedure	Lab Demonstration by Demonstrator		Clinical Demonstration by Student (Verified by Demonstrator)		Remarks
		Date	Signature	Date	Signature	
14	**Use of Restraints**					
	(a) Mummy Restraints					
	(b) Elbow Restraints					
	(c) Clove-hitch Restraints					
	(d) Jacket Restraint					
15	**Assist in Special Procedures**					
	(a) Lumbar Puncture					
	(b) Exchange Transfusion					
	(c) Resuscitation					
	(d) Phototherapy					
16	**Care During Paediatric Emergencies**					
	(a) Asphyxia					
	(b) Convulsions					
	(c) Head Injury					
	(d) Haemolytic Disorders					
17	**Participation in Immunisation Sessions/Camps**					
	Health Teaching					
	(a) Individual					
	(b) Group					

Practical File Work

Nursing Care Plan	Date	Disease condition	Signature
1			
2			
3			
Case Study/Presentation			
1			
2			
Drug Presentation			
1			

Practical Examination

____

Signature of Internal Examiner

Date:

____

Signature of External Examiner

Date:

____

Signature of Internal Examiner

Date:

____

Signature of External Examiner

Date:

Medical Surgical Nursing

S No	Nursing Procedure	Lab Demonstration by Demonstrator		Clinical Demonstration by Student (Verified by Demonstrator)		Remarks
		Date	Signature	Date	Signature	
1	Nursing Assessment • History Taking • Identification of Health Problem					
2	**Preoperative Preparation**					
3	**Postoperative Care**					
	(a) Setting of Postoperative Unit					
	(b) Postoperative Care					
	(c) Surgical Dressing					
	(d) Removal of Sutures					
4	**OT Techniques**					
	General Preparation of OT					
	(a) Surgical Scrubbing					
	(b) Gown and Gloves, Mask					
	(c) Identification of Instruments for Common Surgery					
	(d) Setting up of Trolley for Different Surgeries					

S No	Nursing Procedure	Lab Demonstration by Demonstrator		Clinical Demonstration by Student (Verified by Demonstrator)		Remarks
		Date	Signature	Date	Signature	
	(e) Packing of Drums for Sterilisation: i. Rubber goods ii. Instruments iii. Gloves					
	(f) Endotracheal • Intubation/Suctioning • Extubation					
	(g) Assisting in Major Surgeries					
	1					
	2					
	3					
	(h) Assisting in Minor Surgeries					
	1					
	2					
	3					
5	**Nursing in Intensive Care**					
	(a) Setting up of Emergency Trolley					
	(b) Assisting in ET Intubation					
	(c) Assisting in Suctioning					

S No	Nursing Procedure	Lab Demonstration by Demonstrator		Clinical Demonstration by Student (Verified by Demonstrator)		Remarks
		Date	Signature	Date	Signature	
6	**Neurological Condition**					
	(a) Setting Tray for Neurological Examination					
	(b) Glasgow Coma Scale					
	(c) Care of Patient with Paralysis of Limbs					
	(d) Assisting in Lumbar Puncture					
	(e) Assisting in Ventricular Puncture					
	(f) Cardiopulmonary Resuscitation					
	(g) Preparing Patient for MRI EEG					
7	**Gastrointestinal and Chest Conditions**					
	(a) Assessment of GI System					
	(b) Care of Drainage Tube					
	(c) Care of Colostomy					
	(d) Barium Meal					
	(e) Barium Enema					
	(f) Administration of TPN					

S No	Nursing Procedure	Lab Demonstration by Demonstrator		Clinical Demonstration by Student (Verified by Demonstrator)		Remarks
		Date	Signature	Date	Signature	
8	**Chemical Regulation**					
	(a) Fasting Blood Sugar					
	(b) Postprandial B Sugar					
	(c) Glucose Tolerance Test					
	(d) Administration of Insulin					
	(e) Thyroid Function Test					
9	**Respiratory System**					
	(a) Oxygen Therapy					
	(b) Nebulisation					
	(c) Chest Physiotherapy					
	(d) Cardiopulmonary Resuscitation (BLS)					
10	**Eye/ENT Ward**					
	(a) Instillation of Drops/Ointment					
	• Eye					
	• Ear					
	• Nose					
	(b) Perform Eye Examination					
	(c) Eye Irrigation					
	(d) Preoperative Care of Patient for Eye Surgery					

S No	Nursing Procedure	Lab Demonstration by Demonstrator		Clinical Demonstration by Student (Verified by Demonstrator)		Remarks
		Date	Signature	Date	Signature	
	(e) Care of Patient with Eye Surgeries					
	1					
	2					
	3					
	4					
	5					
	(f) Perform ENT Examinations					
	(g) Ear Irrigation					
	(h) Throat Swab Culture					
	(i) Tracheostomy Care					
	(j) Assist in Removal of Foreign Bodies					
11	**Burns and Scalds**					
	(a) Assessment of Burn Patient					
	(b) Calculate Fluid Requirement of Patient					
	(c) Administration of Fluids and Electrolytes					
	(d) Assist in Burns Dressing					
	(e) Perform Exercise for Burn Patient					

S No	Nursing Procedure	Lab Demonstration by Demonstrator		Clinical Demonstration by Student (Verified by Demonstrator)		Remarks
		Date	Signature	Date	Signature	
12	**Oncology Ward/Unit**					
	(a) Preparation and Assist in Biopsies					
	(b) Assist in Radiotherapy					
	(c) Assist in Chemotherapy					
13	**Musculoskeletal System**					
	(a) Care of Patient with Plaster Cast					
	(b) Care of Patient with Skin Traction					
	(c) Care of Patient with Skeletal Traction					
	(d) Care of Patient with Total Hip/Knee Replacement					

Practical File Work

1 Case Study	Date	Disease Condition	Signature
(a)			
(b)			
2 Nursing Care Plan			
(a)			
(b)			
(c)			
3 Health Talk			
(a)			
(b)			

Practical Examination

Signature of Internal Examiner

Date:

Signature of External Examiner

Date:

Signature of Internal Examiner

Date:

Signature of External Examiner

Date:

Nutrition and Dietetics

S No	Nursing Procedure	Lab Demonstration by Demonstrator		Clinical Demonstration by Student (Verified by Demonstrator)		Remarks
		Date	Signature	Date	Signature	
1	**Preparation of Food for Patient** (a) Liquid Diet (b) Semisolid Diet (c) Solid Diet (d) Low Potassium Diet (e) Low Cholesterol Diet (f) High Calorie Diet (g) High Protein Diet (h) Salt Free Diet (i) Bland Diet					
2	**Therapeutic Diet** (a) Pregnant Woman (b) Diabetic Patient (c) Renal Stones (d) Hypertension (e) Anaemia (f) Fever (g) PEM in Children (h) LBW Baby (i) Nephrotic Syndrome					

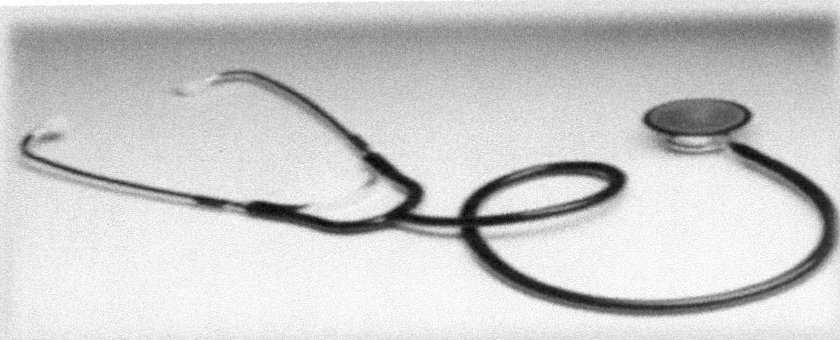

IInd Year Post Basic BSc (Nursing)

Hours of Instruction

Theory: Clinical Experience:

S No	Subjects	Theory (Hours)	Practical (Hours)
1	Sociology	60	–
2	Community Health Nursing	60	240
3	Mental Health Nursing	60	240
4	Introduction to Nursing Education	60	75
5	Introduction to Nursing Administration	60	180
6	Introduction to Nursing Research and Statistics	45	120
	Total	345	855

Subjects and Marks Distributions for Internal Assessment and University Examinations

S No	Subjects	Hours	Internal Assessment	University Exam	Total
1	Sociology	3	25	75	100
2	Community Health Nursing	3	25	75	100
3	Mental Health Nursing	3	25	75	100
4	Introduction to Nursing Education	3	25	75	100
5	Introduction to Nursing Administration	3	25	75	100
6	Introduction to Nursing Research and Statistics*	3	50	–	50
	Practical and Viva Voce				
	• Community Health Nursing		50	50	100
	• Mental Health Nursing		50	50	100
	• Research Project*		50		50

* Research and statistics exam at college level only.

Community Health Nursing

S No	Nursing Procedures	Lab Demonstration by Demonstrator		Clinical Demonstration by Student (Verified by Demonstrator)		Remarks
		Date	Signature	Date	Signature	
1	**Home Visit in Rural and Urban Areas**					
	(a) Community Profile					
	(b) Techniques of IPR					
	(c) Maintaining Health Records					
	(d) Comprehensive Family Health Care					
	(e) Community Health Survey					
2	**Organising and Assisting in**					
	(a) Antenatal and Postnatal Clinic					
	(b) Immunisation					
	(c) Family Welfare Activities					
	(d) School Health Programmes					
	(e) Health Camps					
3	Project Work and Presentation of Reports					
4	**Records**					
	(a) Family Folder					
	(b) Individual					

S No	Nursing Procedures	Lab Demonstration by Demonstrator		Clinical Demonstration by Student (Verified by Demonstrator)		Remarks
		Date	Signature	Date	Signature	
5	**Health Education**					
	(a) Urban					
	(b) Rural					
6	Participate in National Health Programmes					
7	Counselling to Individual, family, Community About HIV, TB, Swine Flu, etc.					
8	Home Visits					
9	Bag Technique					
10	Supervise Health Workers					
11	**Assessment of**					
	(a) Newborn					
	(b) Infant					
	(c) Toddler					
	(d) Preschooler/School Child					
	(e) Adult					
	(f) Antenatal Mother					
	(g) Postnatal Mother					

S No	Nursing Procedures	Lab Demonstration by Demonstrator		Clinical Demonstration by Student (Verified by Demonstrator)		Remarks
		Date	Signature	Date	Signature	
12	**Community Procedures**					
	(a) Performing Handwashing at Home					
	(b) Anthropometric Measurement					
	(c) Urine Analysis					
	(d) Collection of Specimen for Lab Investigation					
	(e) Estimation of Haemoglobin					
	(f) Oral Rehydration Therapy					
	(g) Scabies Treatment					
13	**Visits**					
	(a) School					
	(b) Home for Aged					
	(c) Red Cross Home					
	(d) National Family Planning					
	(e) Epidemic Disease Hospital					
	(f) Water Purification Plant					
	(g) Professional Bodies Like TNAI, PNRC, INC, etc.					
	(h) Industries e.g. Milk, Dairy, etc.					

Comprehensive Health Care

S No	Date	Disease Condition	Signature
1			
2			
3			
4			
5			

Practical Examination

Signature of Internal Examiner

Date:

Signature of External Examiner

Date:

Signature of Internal Examiner

Date:

Signature of External Examiner

Date:

Mental Health Nursing

S No	Nursing Procedure	Lab Demonstration by Demonstrator		Clinical Demonstration by Student (Verified by Demonstrator)		Remarks
		Date	Signature	Date	Signature	
1	Admission and Discharge of Psychiatric Patient					
2	Mental Status Examination					
3	Process Recording					
4	**Nursing Care of Patient with**					
	(a) Psychotic Disorder					
	(b) Neurotic Disorder					
	(c) Organic Conditions					
	(d) Character Disorder					
	(e) Substance Abuse					
5	**Assist in Specific Therapies**					
	(a) ECT					
	(b) Psychotherapy					
	(c) Recreational/Play Therapy					
	(d) Occupational Therapy					
	(e) Milieu Therapy					
	(f) De-Addiction Therapy					

S No	Nursing Procedure	Lab Demonstration by Demonstrator		Clinical Demonstration by Student (Verified by Demonstrator)		Remarks
		Date	Signature	Date	Signature	
	(g) Behavioural Therapy					
	(h) Therapeutic Touch/Massage					
6	Administration of Psychotherapeutic Drugs					
7	**Counselling**					
	(a) Premarital					
	(b) Marital					
	(c) Genetic					
	(d) Individual					
	(e) Group					
	(f) Family					
8	Crisis Intervention					
9	**Community Psychiatry**					
	(a) Conduct Case Study					
	(b) Identify Person with Mental Health Illness					
	(c) Assist in Mental Health Camps					

Nursing Care Plans

S No	Date	Disease condition	Signature
1			
2			
3			
4			
5			

Practical Examination

Signature of Internal Examiner

Date:

Signature of External Examiner

Date:

Signature of Internal Examiner

Date:

Signature of External Examiner

Date:

Introduction to Nursing Education

S No	Nursing Procedure	Lab Demonstration by Demonstrator		Clinical Demonstration by Student (Verified by Demonstrator)		Remarks
		Date	Signature	Date	Signature	
1	**Preparation of Teaching Aids**					
	(a) Lesson Plan					
	(b) Charts					
	(c) Posters					
	(d) Flash Cards					
	(e) Leaflets					
	(f) Pamphlet					
	(g) Model					
	(h) Bulletin Board					
	(i) Transparencies					
	(j) Powerpoint					
2	Preparation of Master Rotation Plan					
3	Preparation of Evaluation Tools					
4	Role Play					

Classroom Teachings

S No	Topic	Date	Supervised by
1			
2			

Introduction to Nursing Research and Statistics

Note: Group of students have option to select the Research Project in their area of interest in the beginning of IInd year with their respective supervisors

Title of the Research Project : ______________________

____

____

____

____

Date of Submission of Report : ______________________

Date of Presentations : ______________________

Signature of Supervisor : ______________________

Signature of Co-supervisor : ______________________

Signature of the Principal : ______________________

Basic Important Formulas

1. Conversion Formulas

i. Conversion of Fahrenheit scale to Celsius scale

$$C = (F - 32) \times \frac{5}{9}$$

ii. Conversion of Celsius scale to Fahrenheit scale

$$F = (C \times \frac{9}{5}) + 32$$

iii. Inches to centimetre

1 Inch = 2.54 cm

1 cm = 0.39 inch

iv. Minim to millilitre

1 minim = 0.06 ml

1 ml = 15 minims

v. Equivalent imperical and metric quantities

1 gram	=	65 miligrams
1 ounce	=	28 grams
1 pound	=	453 grams
2.2 pound	=	1 Kg
1 table spoon	=	3 tea spoon = 15 ml
1 teacup	=	150 – 180 ml
1 standard glass	=	240 – 250 ml
1 ounce	=	30 ml
1 pound	=	16 ounces
1 Kg	=	2.2 pounds
1 drop	=	1/20 ml or 0.05 ml
1 pint	=	500 ml

2. **Important Formulas**

i. Bod Mass Index (BMI)

$$\text{BMI} = \frac{\text{Weight in Kg}}{\text{Height in meter square}}$$

ii. Dosage calculation in children

(a) According to Body Surface Area

$$\text{Child's dose} = \frac{\text{Child's body surface area}}{\text{Adult's body surface area}} \times \text{Adult dose}$$

(b) Young's Formula

According to Age

$$\text{Child's dose} = \frac{\text{Age of child}}{\text{Age + 12}} \times \text{Adult dose}$$

(c) Clark's Formula

According to Body Weight

$$\text{Child's dose} = \frac{\text{Weight of child in pounds}}{150} \times \text{Adult dose}$$

3. **Calculation of Flow Rate**

$$\text{Drop/Minute} = \frac{\text{Total volume to be infused}}{\text{Time in minutes}} \times \text{Drop factor}$$

Drop factor

Micro drip set

60 drops = 1 ml

Macro drip set

16 drops = 1 ml

4. Infusion Time Calculation

$$\text{Infusion Time} = \frac{\text{Total volume to be infused}}{\text{Ml per hour to be infused}}$$

5. Expected Date of Delivery (EDD)

EDD = Date of LMP + 9 months + 7 days

6. Percentage of Malnutrition

$$\text{\% age of malnutrition} = \frac{\text{Actual weight}}{\text{Expected weight}} \times 100$$

7. Formula for Calculating Expected Weight

(a) For Age (1 month to 12 months)

$$\text{Weight} = \frac{\text{Age in months}}{2} + 9$$

(b) For Age (1–6 years)

Weight = (Age in years × 2) + 8

(c) For Age (6–12 years)

$$\text{Weight} = \frac{(\text{Age in years} \times 9)}{2} - 5$$

8. Important facts

(a) Normal birth weight of Indian newborn = 2.5–3 Kg

(b) Birth weight doubles by age of 5–6 months

(c) Birth weight triples by age of 1 year

(d) Birth weight becomes 4 times at age of 2 years, five times at age of 3 years and 10 times by 10 years

9. Calculation of Height

a) At birth is approx = 45–55 cm
b) At 1 year of age = About 75 cm
c) At 1–12 years of age

Height = (Age in years × 6) + 77 cm

10. Inteligence Quotient Calculation Formula

$$\text{IQ} = \frac{\text{Mental age}}{\text{Chronological age}} \times 100 \text{ or } = \frac{\text{MA}}{\text{CA}} \times 100$$

Fluid Requirement for Newborn Baby and Paediatric Clients

Formulas for calculating Fluid and Electrolyte Requirement for Paediatric clients

Holiday Segar Method

Up to 10 kg	:	100 ml/kg/day
11 – 20 kg	:	1000 ml + 50 ml/kg/day above 10 kg
21 kg onwards:		1500 ml + 20 to 25 ml/kg/day for extra weight

Sodium	:	3 – 4 meq/kg/day
Potassium	:	2 – 3 meq/kg/day
Chloride	:	3 – 4 meq/kg/day

For Example: A baby weighing 8.5 Kg will require fluid as

$8.5 \times 100 = 850$ ml/day

13 Kg weight will require

$(10\times 100) + (50 \times 3) = 1150$ ml

22 Kg Body weight will require

$(10 \times 100) + (10 \times 50) + (2 \times 20) = 1540$ ml/day

Types of fluids commonly used in Paediatric Area

- At birth, For the first 2 days – Dextrose 5% or 10%
- After that, for preterm babies – N/5 in 10% dextrose
- For term babies – N/5 in 5% dextrose
- For 3–6 months – N/4 in 5% dextrose
- At 6 months – N/3 in 5% dextrose
- After 5 years – NS or 5% dextrose

Useful Normal Laboratory Values

Blood Serum

	Normal Value
Bleeding Time	1–3 minutes
Clotting Time	3–10 minutes
Erythrocyte Sedimentation Rate	< 20–30 mm/hr
Platelet Count	2,00,000 – 4,50,000/cumm
Haemoglobin	Females : 12–16 gm/dl Male : 14–16 gm/dl
WBC Count	5000–10,000 cumm
Neutrophills	40–75%
Eosinophills	1–6%
Basophills	0–1%
Lymphocytes	20–45%
Monocytes	2–10%
Reticulocytes	0.2%
Blood Sugar (Fasting)	60–100 mg/dl
Blood Sugar PP/Random	120–150 mg/dl
Blood Urea	10–40 mg/dl
Serum Creatinine	0.5–1.4 mg/dl
Serum Cholestrol	130–250 mg/dl
Serum Bilirubin(Total)	0.2–1.0 mg/dl
Serum Bilirubin (Direct)	0.0–0.2 mg/dl
Serum Bilirubin (Indirect)	0.2–0.8 mg/dl
Uric Acid	2.5–7.0 mg/dl
Calcium	8.8–10.8 mg/dl
Sodium	135–145 meq/dl
Phosphorus	1.5–6.5 mg/dl
Chloride	90–107 meq/dl
Total Protein	6.3–8.3 gm/dl
Albumin	3.5–5.5 gm/dl
SGOT	4–40 μ/l
SGPT	5– 45 μ/l
Triglycerides	40–160 mg/dl
Total Lipids	400–700 mg/dl
PH Value	7.35–7.45 (Adult)

Urine Output at Different Ages

S No	Age	Normal Urine Output (ml/24hour)
1	Newborn	250
2	2 months	450
3	1 year	500
4	2 years	550
5	4 years	650
6	7 years	750
7	11 years	1100
8	14 years	1200
9	Adult	1500

Clinical Posting for the Post Basic BSc Nursing Students

Month	First Year	Second Year
August		
September		
October		
November		
December		
January		
February		
March		
April		
May		
June		
July		

Signature of the Class Coordinator
Date:

Signature of the Principal
Date: